# Your Marriage Success Guide: Cracking the Code to Lasting Love!

Earl R. Jones

Introduction

# INTRODUCTION

**Marriage is not rainbows and butterflies**

Marriage is a perplexing and complex foundation that includes different difficulties and real factors past the underlying energy and sentiment. While it may very well be a wellspring of satisfaction, love, and happiness, it is critical to recognize that marriage isn't generally portrayed by consistent joy and straightforwardness.

As a general rule, relationships frequently require exertion, split the difference, and viable correspondence to explore through troubles and clashes. Couples might confront conflicts, contrasts in feelings, and different life stressors that can strain the relationship. Monetary issues, vocation requests, nurturing liabilities, and self-awareness can likewise influence the elements inside a marriage.

It is urgent to perceive that keeping a sound and effective marriage requires responsibility, understanding, and the eagerness to deal with difficulties together. This might include looking for proficient assistance, like couples treatment, to resolve fundamental issues and further develop correspondence.

While it is normal to want an amicable and ecstatic organization, it is essential to have reasonable assumptions and comprehend that marriage includes both high points and low points. By recognizing and tending to the intricacies of marriage, couples can fabricate a more grounded establishment and explore through the unavoidable difficulties that emerge, eventually encouraging a more profound and seriously satisfying relationship.

Marriage is much of the time portrayed as not rainbows and butterflies , implying that it isn't generally a smooth and easy excursion. This expression underscores the truth that marriage includes difficulties, and compromises that couples should explore together.

One of the fundamental motivations behind why marriage isn't generally a walk in the park is the intrinsic contrasts between people. Every individual brings their own special foundations, convictions, values, and assumptions into the relationship. These distinctions can prompt contentions, mistaken assumptions, and conflicts, which require open correspondence and split the difference to determine.

Moreover, outer factors, for example, monetary tensions, profession requests, and family obligations can add pressure to a marriage. Adjusting work-life responsibilities, overseeing funds, and bringing up kids can strain the relationship and require cautious exchange and cooperation.

# CHAPTER 1

## The Truth About Happy Marriages

Blissful relationships are based on an underpinning of affection, trust, and common regard. They include a profound close to home association and a promise to support and sustain each other's development and prosperity. Nonetheless, it is critical to comprehend that blissful relationships are not without any trace of difficulties or clashes.

Actually, cheerful relationships require exertion, correspondence, and split the difference from the two accomplices. Couples should pay attention to one another, see each other's requirements and points of view, and work together to track down answers for issues. This includes compelling relational abilities, compassion, and the capacity to determine clashes in a solid and valuable way.

Blissful relationships likewise include a feeling of shared values and objectives. Couples who have a comparable vision for their future and are adjusted in their needs will quite often have a more grounded bond. They support each other's singular yearnings and work together towards shared objectives, whether it's structure of a family, chasing after vocations, or self-awareness.

One more significant part of blissful relationships is the capacity to keep a feeling of closeness and association. This incorporates actual closeness, profound closeness, and hanging out. Couples who focus on getting to know one another, taking part in shared exercises, and communicating love will quite often have additional satisfying connections.

It is significant that cheerful relationships are not static. They require continuous exertion and flexibility as people and conditions change after some time. Couples should develop and advance together, changing in accordance with new jobs, obligations, and life stages.

Couples who are blissful or if nothing else is fulfilled in their relationship can have contrasts in characters, leisure activities and family values. They can squabble about exactly the same things as despondent couples do, like cash, kids, sex, family errands and the parents in law. While no two relationships are similar, the exploration led at Washington State College by Dr John Gottman found that cheerful couples followed a similar arrangement of seven standards - regardless of whether they know it. These standards start with building a profound fellowship, then, at that point, battling reasonably and finally making a significant relationship with expectation. The individuals who were unsettled typically missed the mark concerning at least one of the standards.

Cheerful relationships are somewhat flawed using any and all means, the fact of the matter is no relationship is blissful constantly. In any case, the relationships that are blissful had the option to keep a profound kinship in any event, during struggle. All in all, they were being good to one another - in any event, when they were clashing.

Moreover, over the long haul, couples might encounter changes in their sentiments, needs, and self-improvement. This can prompt changes in elements inside the marriage and require continuous work to adjust and keep areas of strength for it.

It is critical to take note that the difficulties in marriage don't suggest that it is ill-fated to fizzle or be miserable. Rather, they feature the requirement for sensible assumptions and a promise to manage hardships together. Fruitful relationships require powerful correspondence, compassion, understanding, and an eagerness to think twice about.

Cheerful couples are two individuals who are benevolent to one another, realize each other well and express their affection through little motions as a feature of their everyday lives. They assume the best about one another. They understand what their accomplice likes and needs and attempt to give it or assist their joint forces with accomplishing it however much they can. They pay special attention to one another in little and huge ways. They actually have struggles and can fly off the handle, the key with cheerful couples is that they are helpful in their contention. They work to keep up with positive ways of behaving like clarifying pressing issues or staying sympathetic during a conflict.

At last, reality with regards to cheerful relationships is that they are a consequence of nonstop venture, responsibility, and the readiness to explore difficulties together. While no marriage is great, couples who focus on open correspondence, common regard, and shared values have a higher probability of encountering enduring satisfaction and satisfaction in their relationship.

# CHAPTER 2

## Marital Conflict

Conjugal struggles are conflicts or strains between companions inside a marriage. They can emerge from different sources, including correspondence breakdowns, contrasts in values, monetary issues, nurturing styles, and outer stressors. These struggles might appear in changed structures, like contentions, close to home distance, or even actual articulations of disappointment.

Correspondence breakdowns frequently assume a critical part, as misinterpretations or an absence of successful correspondence can raise minor issues into bigger struggles. Contrasts in assumptions, requirements, or objectives can likewise contribute, prompting sensations of disappointment or hatred. Monetary strains are one more typical wellspring of contention, where conflicts over spending, saving, or monetary needs can make pressure.

In marriage, struggle happens when the requirements and wants of companions wander and are consequently contradictory. Since mates connect with one another in regards to various issues vital to their marriage over the long haul, unavoidable struggle will happen somewhat in each marriage at any rate. It isn't the presence of contention in marriage fundamentally that is unfavorable to conjugal fulfillment or soundness, yet the way in which mates oversee struggle when it happens. Clashes can be settled emphatically through conversation, yet now and again may bring about the heightening of contending without goal, or with every companion overlooking the area of contention trying to forestall negative conjugal communications. The nature of the marriage endures when clashes stay unsettled, and in a relationship the powerlessness to effectively oversee struggle can prompt actual maltreatment, at times with extreme results.

All couples have contentions about things yet there are a few contentions that are more normal than others. Repeating contentions negatively affect connections and can possibly debase and obliterate the relationship. The three most normal contexts with couples are about sex, cash, and kids.

- Sex: This is likely the most successive wellspring of contention between couples. Frequently there are conflicts about the recurrence of sex with one individual inclination their necessities are not being met and the other individual inclination pestered or baited. A few couples quarrel over who does the starting, the absence of foreplay, sexual position, or sexual demonstrations. Most contentions are driven by contrasts in needs, requirements, inclinations, and sex drive or charisma. Basically this contention is the couples battle with correspondence and knowing how to explore towards exchange and split the difference.

- Cash: The issues connected with cash that couples squabble over are various and many. Models incorporate what to burn through cash on, the amount to save, what we are putting something aside for, needs versus needs, whether to blend cash or keep it isolated, how bills ought to be separated and paid for, how to make a spending plan, or what ought to be remembered for the financial plan. Clashes can possibly occur when cash is running low, couples are straying into the red, quarreling over how to escape obligation, or who is answerable for the obligations. Seldom do couples totally agree to cash the board, objectives, methodologies, or cycles.

- Kids: The last subject couples are particularly energetic about are youngsters. Many couples end up contending even before they have youngsters. They might quarrel over whether to have them, when to have them, the number of to have, names, thus substantially more. In some cases there are contentions while attempting to get pregnant particularly in the event that there are issues with ripeness and choosing how much the couple will go to have a kid. When kids show up an entirely different arrangement of potential contentions crop up, for example, who will get up with the youngster in the center evening, whether one parent ought to remain at home to bring up the kid, what to take care of them, how to dress them, nurturing, and disciplinary measures, level of checking and oversight, thus significantly more.

- Others: In spite of the fact that sex, cash, and kids are the main three things couples squabble over, there are a few other ordinarily happening issues with couples. A portion of the other normal subjects couples quarrel over are divisions of work, parents in law, the planning of life altering situations, quality time together, annoyances, envy, companions, correspondence, work, control, and legislative issues.

Conjugal contentions can affect the close to home prosperity of the two accomplices and the general dependability of the relationship. It's fundamental for couples to address clashes productively, cultivating open correspondence, sympathy, and split the difference. Looking for proficient assistance, like couples treatment, can be useful in exploring and settling further issues.

Seeing each other's points of view, rehearsing undivided attention, and figuring out some mutual interest are critical stages in overseeing conjugal contentions and cultivating a solid, enduring relationship.

# CHAPTER 3

**Solve your problems**

Taking care of conjugal issues includes successful correspondence, understanding, and a readiness to cooperate. Here are a moves toward help address and resolve issues in your marriage:

1. Open Correspondence: Talk about your interests straightforwardly and genuinely with your accomplice. Obviously express your sentiments, necessities, and viewpoints while effectively paying

attention to your accomplice's considerations too.

2. Undivided attention: Focus on your accomplice's sentiments and concerns. Reflecting back what you've heard can guarantee that both of you see each other's viewpoints.

3. Compassion: Attempt to figure out your accomplice's perspective, regardless of whether you concur. Compassion makes an association and cultivates a more helpful environment.

4. Pick the Perfect Opportunity: Timing matters. Pick a quiet and proper opportunity to examine issues as opposed to tending to them without giving it much thought.

5. Keep away from Fault: Spotlight on the issue instead of accusing one another. Use "I" articulations to communicate your

sentiments and necessities without blaming your accomplice.

6. Look for Split the difference: track down center ground and split the difference. It's really not necessary to focus on one individual winning and the other losing, yet tracking down arrangements that work for both of you.

7. Set Practical Assumptions: Comprehend that no relationship is awesome. Set reasonable assumptions and know that clashes are a characteristic piece of any organization.

8. Think about Proficient Assistance: In the event that issues continue to happen or are especially difficult, looking for the assistance of an expert, like a couples specialist, can give direction and backing.

9. Quality Time Together: Reinforce your association by getting to know one

another. Take part in exercises that you both appreciate to support the positive parts of your relationship.

10. Center around Arrangements, Not Issues: Rather than harping exclusively on the issues, effectively cooperate to track down reasonable arrangements. This cooperative methodology can assist with building a more grounded starting point for your relationship.

Keep in mind, each marriage is special, and the viability of these techniques might fluctuate. Persistence, understanding, and a guarantee to cooperating are fundamental parts of settling conjugal issues.

# CHAPTER 4

**Building trust and respect**

Trust is an irreplaceable fixing in building and keeping a solid marriage. Confiding in each other is one of the main components of your relationship, and a significant component of any lifetime responsibility. Without trust, the nature of your relationship will fall apart.

A relationship that needs trust is a relationship in trouble. On the off chance that trust is absent in a marriage or relationship it is beyond the realm of possibilities for the relationship to flourish.

Building trust and regard in a relationship is a continuous cycle that requires steady exertion from the two accomplices. Here are a few key techniques:

- Transparent Correspondence: Cultivate straightforwardness by transparently sharing your contemplations and sentiments. Be a decent audience and urge your accomplice to communicate their thoughts unafraid of judgment.

- Dependability: Stay true to your obligations and responsibilities. Reliably finishing what you say assembles trust over the long run.

- Consistency: Exhibit dependability and consistency in your activities. This makes a feeling that all is well with the world in the relationship.

- Regard Limits: Recognize and regard your accomplice's very own limits. Laying out and respecting these limits fabricates trust and shows that you esteem and value one another.

- Apologize and Pardon: When missteps occur, apologize genuinely. Similarly significant is the capacity to pardon. Clutching hard feelings dissolves trust and regard.

- Sympathy: Comprehend and approve your accomplice's sentiments. Show sympathy by imagining their perspective and exhibiting that you care about their encounters.

- Shared Values: Recognize and build up shared values that structure the groundwork of your relationship. Normal qualities make a feeling of solidarity and common comprehension.

- Support One another: Show up for your accomplice in both great and testing times. Offering help builds up the possibility that you are a solid and caring presence in their life.

- Concede Errors: Nobody is awesome. Conceding when you're off-base exhibits lowliness and a promise to genuineness.

- Quality Time: Hang out to develop your association. This can be just about as basic as getting a charge out of shared exercises or having significant discussions.

- Observe Accomplishments: Recognize and commend each other's accomplishments, both of all shapes and sizes. Uplifting feedback fortifies the connection between accomplices.

Recollect that building trust and regard is a continuous interaction. It requires persistence, understanding, and a certified obligation to the prosperity of the relationship. Routinely check in with one another to guarantee that you are both feeling appreciated, comprehended, and esteemed.

# CHAPTER 5

## Maintaining Physical and Emotional Intimacy

Intimacy in a relationship is a sensation of being close, and genuinely associated and upheld. It implies having the option to share an entire scope of considerations, sentiments and encounters that we have as individuals. It includes being open and talking through your viewpoints and feelings, letting your watchman down (being defenseless), and showing another person how you feel and what your deepest desires are.

Intimacy is developed after some time, and it requires persistence and exertion from the two accomplices to make and keep up with. Finding closeness with somebody you love can be one of the most compensating parts of a relationship.

Aside from profound and sexual closeness, you can likewise be cozy mentally, casually, monetarily, profoundly, innovatively (for instance, remodeling your home) and on occasion of emergency (filling in collectively during difficult stretches).

Closeness is accomplished when we become near another person and are consoled that we are adored and acknowledged for what our identity is. Youngsters ordinarily foster closeness with guardians and friends. As grown-ups, we look for closeness in cozy associations with different grown-ups, companions, family and with an accomplice.

Keeping up with actual closeness includes open correspondence, focusing on quality time, and being mindful of one another's requirements. Close to home closeness requires trust, weakness, and undivided attention. Routinely communicating adoration and appreciation reinforces the two parts of a marriage.

Keeping up with physical and profound closeness in a marriage is pivotal for a sound and satisfying relationship. Here is a complete gander at the two perspectives:

## Physical Intimacy

Correspondence: Straightforwardly talk about wants, inclinations, and worries to guarantee common comprehension.

Share dreams and investigate better approaches to keep the actual association energetic.

Quality Time: Focus on time together without interruptions to reinforce the profound bond, which emphatically influences actual closeness.

Sentiment; Keep the sentiment alive through signals like astonishment date evenings, smart gifts, or love notes.

Variety: Explore various parts of actual closeness to forestall routine and weariness.

Wellbeing and Taking care of oneself: Urge each other to keep up with actual prosperity, as it straightforwardly impacts one's capacity to participate in cozy exercises.

Versatility: Be available to adjust to changes in actual closeness because of life stages, medical problems, or different variables.


## Emotional Intimacy

Trust: Construct and keep up with trust through genuineness, unwavering quality, and keeping guarantees.

Weakness: Offer sentiments, fears, and dreams straightforwardly, making a profound close to home association.

Undivided attention: Practice mindful paying attention to see each other's feelings and concerns.

Compassion: Come at the situation from your accomplice's perspective, showing sympathy during both blissful and testing times.

Compromise: Foster sound compromise abilities to address conflicts without harming profound closeness.

Warmth and Appreciation: Consistently express love and appreciation for one another to build up profound bonds.

Shared Objectives: Lay out and make progress toward shared objectives, cultivating a feeling of organization and solidarity.

Quality Correspondence: Past sharing everyday encounters, take part in more profound discussions about values, yearnings, and self-improvement.

Advising: Look for proficient assistance if necessary, as treatment can give instruments to upgrade profound closeness.

In rundown, an effective marriage includes a unique exchange among physical and close to home closeness. By supporting these viewpoints, couples can make major areas of strength for an enduring and satisfying relationship.

# CHAPTER 6

**Balancing Work, Family And Marriage**

Adjusting work, family, and marriage includes focusing on liabilities and overseeing time successfully. Correspondence is vital; examine assumptions with your mate and lay out a steady climate. Put down sensible objectives and stopping points to keep away from overcommitting. Focus on quality time with family, and timetable ordinary exercises together. Figure out how to appoint assignments at work and home, and embrace adaptability to adjust to evolving conditions. Taking care of oneself is fundamental; distribute time for individual prosperity to support a solid balance between fun and serious activities. Routinely rethink and change your methodology as conditions develop.

Adjusting work and day to day life can be really difficult for any hitched couple. It means a lot to figure out how to adjust both so that each accomplice can feel upheld and satisfied in their jobs. This article will give a few hints on the most proficient method to adjust work and everyday life in marriage.

Work and everyday life can be challenging to adjust to. All couples should figure out how to adjust their work and home life, while as yet possessing energy for one another. This is particularly valid for hitched couples who have youngsters. Shuffling work, home, and family requests can be distressing, yet with a couple of tips and systems, wedded couples can figure out how to track down an equilibrium that works for them.

## GET TO KNOW ONE ANOTHER

Investing quality energy with your life partner is fundamental for a solid marriage. Focus on it to plan ordinary date evenings and ends of the week from work and family obligations. Set aside some margin to talk, tune in, and appreciate each other's conversation.

## SHARE LIABILITIES

Sharing liabilities can assist with decreasing pressure and take a portion of the strain of working guardians. Talk about how you can split liabilities, like childcare, housework, and tasks so you both similarly share the heap.

## MAKE A FAMILY SCHEDULE

Making a family schedule can assist with guaranteeing that everybody in the family knows about forthcoming occasions and obligations. This permits every individual to prepare and ensure that there is sufficient time for both work and family. It can likewise assist with lessening pressure by ensuring that all relatives know about what is generally anticipated from them and when.

## SET ASIDE A FEW MINUTES FOR YOURSELF

Setting aside a few minutes for yourself is a significant piece of adjusting work and day to day life. It is essential to require an investment for yourself every day to accomplish something that you appreciate like perusing, working out, or going for a stroll. This can assist with lessening pressure and can assist with making balance in your life.

# CHAPTER 7

## Overcoming Struggles And Adversities

Beating battles and misfortunes in marriage includes a mix of correspondence, versatility, and common help. Transparent correspondence is pivotal to seeing each other's viewpoints and tracking down arrangements. Building strength as a team includes adjusting to difficulties and gaining from encounters as opposed to allowing them to characterize the relationship adversely.

Shared help incorporates being there for one another inwardly, genuinely, and intellectually during troublesome times. Looking for proficient direction, for example, marriage mentoring, can likewise give important experiences and instruments to exploring difficulties together. At last, areas of strength for an is based on an underpinning of trust, sympathy, and the common obligation to enduring life's difficulties collectively.

Conquering battles and difficulties in marriage requires a proactive and cooperative methodology. Here are exhaustive moves toward explore difficulties:

- Open Correspondence: Encourage a climate where the two accomplices have a solid sense of security offering their viewpoints and feelings. Plan customary registrations to talk about worries, objectives, and sentiments.

- Undivided attention: Practice undivided attention by completely thinking, understanding, answering, and recollecting what your accomplice shares.

Try not to hinder and show sympathy towards their viewpoint.

- Sympathy and Understanding: Come at the situation from your accomplice's perspective to more readily grasp their sentiments and perspective.

Recognize each other's encounters without judgment.

- Shared Regard: Approach each other with deference even in the midst of conflict.

Stay away from individual assaults and spotlight on the main thing.

- Group Mindset: Move toward difficulties collectively, underscoring that the two accomplices are pursuing a shared objective.

Share liabilities and work together on tracking down arrangements.

- Set Practical Assumptions: Perceive that no relationship is great, and difficulties are a characteristic piece of marriage.

Change assumptions and be adaptable in adjusting to evolving conditions.

- Critical thinking Abilities: Cooperate to recognize the main drivers of issues. Conceptualize and execute reasonable arrangements, zeroing in on split the difference and participation.

- Look for Proficient Assistance: Consider marriage mentoring or treatment to acquire experiences from a nonpartisan outsider. Proficient direction can give devices and procedures to settling clashes.

- Self-Reflection: Assess your own decisions and commitments to clashes. Roll out private improvements to assist the relationship.

- Quality Time: Devote time to support the close to home association by taking part in exercises you both appreciate and build up the positive parts of your relationship.

- Emergency as a Chance for Development: View difficulties as any open doors for individual and social development. Gain from previous encounters to reinforce the marriage pushing ahead.

- Tolerance and Determination: Comprehend that settling issues might require some investment.

Remain focused on the interaction and show restraint toward one another.

By joining these methodologies, couples can fabricate flexibility, fortify their bond, and beat the battles and afflictions that might emerge in marriage.

# CONCLUSION

The significance of correspondence in marriage is much of the time not treated in a serious way as many couples will generally imagine that the day to day talk or its absence doesn't influence them on an everyday premise. Be that as it may, correspondence is the vehicle through which any remaining significant pieces of marriage are performed.

Love, trust, genuineness, and each and every significant quality of a solid marriage aren't significant in themselves. The statement of these things creates a marriage worth begrudging.
Showing that adoration, displaying your trust, and acting sincerely is where the enchantment is. Having the option to convey how much your significant other or spouse means to you is where your marriage goes from great to incredible..